# Bath Salts

# Basics

I0417509

*Easy Guide to Homemade Bath Salts*

*Including Simple Recipes*

By: Stella Bright

## Disclaimer & Terms of Use

Effort has been made to ensure that the information in this book is accurate and complete, however, the author and the publisher do not warrant the accuracy of the information, text, and graphics contained within the book due to the rapidly changing nature of science, research, known and unknown facts and internet. The Author and the publisher do not hold any responsibility for errors, omissions or contrary interpretation of the subject matter herein. This book is presented solely for motivational and informational purposes only.

The recipes and information provided in this report are for educational purposes only and are not intended to provide medical advice. Readers are strongly encouraged to consult a

# Contents

Copyright © 2015/Stella Bright ...........................................2

Disclaimer & Terms of Use ...............................................2

INTRODUCTION ...............................................................7

THE SALTS AND KEY BENEFITS ........................................ 10

    Sea Salt ................................................................ 11

    Epsom Salt ........................................................... 11

    Dead Sea Mineral Salt............................................ 12

    Himalayan Pink Salt .............................................. 12

THE LIQUID OILS AND KEY BENEFITS ........................... 13

    Avocado Oil .......................................................... 14

    Almond Oil ........................................................... 14

    Jojoba Oil ............................................................. 15

    Neem Oil............................................................... 15

    Walnut Oil............................................................. 16

    Apricot Kernel Oil.................................................. 16

    Hazelnut Oil.......................................................... 17

Grape Seed Oil............................................................17

Olive Oil....................................................................17

THE ESSENTIAL OILS & KEY BENEFITS ...............................18

Lavender Oil ..............................................................19

Eucalyptus Oil ...........................................................19

Rosemary Oil .............................................................19

Peppermint Oil ..........................................................20

Grapefruit Oil ............................................................20

Rose Oil ....................................................................20

Tea tree ....................................................................21

Vanilla Oil..................................................................21

Lemon Oil..................................................................21

PREPARATION STORAGE & USE OF BATH SALTS...................22

Preparing Bath Salts ...................................................23

Storing Bath Salts .......................................................25

USING BATH SALTS......................................................28

SIMPLE BATH SALT RECIPES ...............................................29

Glow Salt Recipe ............................................................ 30

Neem Chamomile & Dried Flowers.................................. 31

Salt Scrub by Dead Sea Salts .......................................... 32

Crystal Salt .................................................................... 33

Milky Bath Salt............................................................... 34

Lavender Bath Salt ......................................................... 35

Aromatherapy Pink Bath Salt........................................... 36

Vanilla Epsom Bath Salt .................................................. 37

Aromatherapy Almond Bath Salt...................................... 38

Eucalyptus Bath Salts...................................................... 39

Energizer Bath Salt ......................................................... 40

Back Pain Relaxing Bath Salts.......................................... 41

Before you go….. ............................................................ 42

# INTRODUCTION

Your skin is your largest organ. What you put on your skin is absorbed into your tissues and your circulatory system. It is vital that what is placed on your skin is something you <u>choose</u> to put into your body. Products that are natural hold key benefits to our body, mind, and soul, and are essential in the ever-connected world in which we live.

Making therapeutic bath salts is quite simple. Bath salts are a wonderful way to implement aromatherapy, skin care, and healing benefits. To me, there is nothing better than a long hot soak in a lightly scented bath. I have been known to complete my daily meditation in the tub!

Bath Salts are prepared from an alkaline base that is able to neutralize the acids present on the skin. As salts are capable of increasing the salinity of water, they tend to lower the bacteria count on your skin. Bath salts mixed with essential oils provide a fragrance that clings to the body long after you emerge from the bath. While the salts are healing and relaxing, the scents are comforting, and the carrier oils are hydrating. Taking a warm bath in these salted scents not only cleanses you, but the bath will also refresh and relax you. A scented salt bath is a refuge from the robotic, stressful, modern life.

Making these salts at home is a decadent luxury that is deliciously affordable.

Homemade and tailored to your personal desires, bath salts are the treasures you can relish every day. This book is intended to help the reader by providing an insight of basic Bath Salts, their ingredients, preparation, storage, and the healing recipes. You can find different kinds of salts and liquid oils available in the market today, but it can be difficult to choose the right ingredients. Let me help you choose the best combination of these salts and oils depending on your needs and specifications by providing you the basic knowledge of the salts, liquid oils, and the essential oils.

Benefits of bathing with these scented salty treasures are:

- Aiding your skin with exfoliation.

- Soothing dry irritated skin and moisturizes the skin.

- Essential oils provide fragrance that can increase energy and elevate your mood.

- Naturally occurring minerals, like potassium and magnesium, can increase your metabolism and decrease high blood pressure.

- Salts can wick away water bloat and reduce swelling and inches.

- Soothing muscles from sports injury or overuse.

# THE SALTS AND KEY BENEFITS

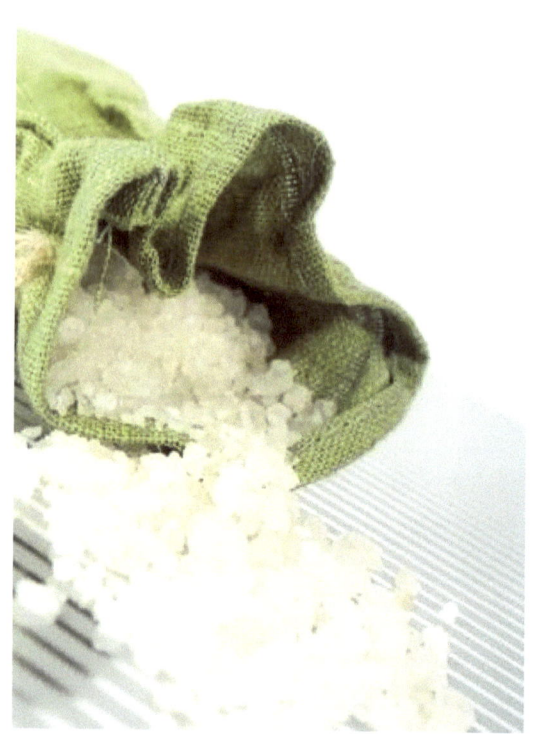

The base salts are the most important ingredient of any Bath Salt Recipe and there are a great variety of choices available. Each salt has its own unique look and therapeutic properties.

## Sea Salt

Sea Salt contains around 97% sodium chloride, which is the chemical used in preparation of table salt but unlike table salt, sea salt contains various other salts too. The constituents depend on where the salt comes from as different seas have different concentration of these minerals. Sea Salt is well known for its therapeutic properties and health enhancing minerals. Adding just a little Sea Salt to the bath can ease muscle cramps, stimulate circulation, and soothe overworked achy legs and feet.

## Epsom Salt

Epsom Salt is chemically Magnesium Sulphate. It is known for centuries for its tranquil properties. It is a classic bath salt that helps in reducing the inflammation on the skin and hence, it has been used historically as a soak for tired muscles and aches. It soothes various types of skin problems, such as acne and infections. People who are deficient in Magnesium are advised to bath in Epsom Salt for about 20 minutes as the body absorbs Magnesium through the skin. It is believed to increase relaxation by raising the serotonin levels and improves the mood by lowering adrenaline and stress.

## Dead Sea Mineral Salt

Dead Sea Mineral Salt is quite different from other sea salts as it is land-locked and the levels of salts are ten times more concentrated than in oceans. It is only about 15% Sodium Chloride, unlike regular sea salt. Dead Sea Salt is known for its therapeutic properties since ancient times and is used today to treat skin conditions and arthritis.

## Himalayan Pink Salt

The Himalayan Pink Salt, as the name suggests, comes from the Himalayan Mountains and is a shade of pink. Having formed underground in ancient times, Himalayan Pink Salt is quite ancient and pure. The pink shade is due to its iron content. The salt has been used for centuries for healing purpose. It also stimulates the blood flow, lowers blood pressure, soothes tired muscles, removes toxins and decreases the acid influx.

# THE LIQUID OILS AND KEY BENEFITS

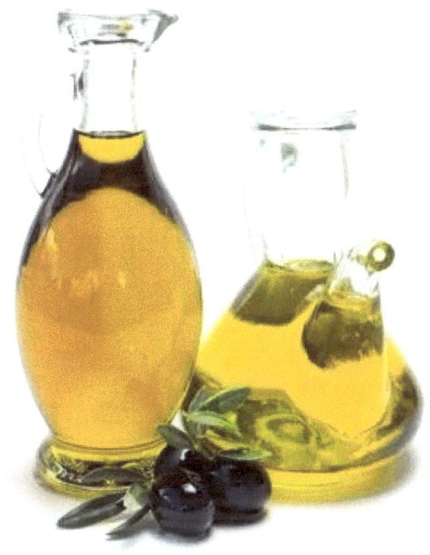

Blending salts with liquid oils is a wonderful synergistic combination. Relaxing properties of hot water compliment the effect of well-chosen salts and liquid oils. Aromatic baths created with these and scrubs can provide relief from stress, unease and assist with muscular and joint pains. It is also beneficial in treating severe skin conditions.

## Avocado Oil

This oil is very rich in antioxidants and especially Vitamin E. These two ingredients are known to be a very powerful helper in the battle against skin aging, protecting skin cells from oxidation, and fighting free radicals. Avocado Oil protects the skin from harmful UV rays therefore decreasing the chances of being burned by the sun, reducing the risk of skin cancer and preventing the appearance of age spots. It is said to aid in wound healing.

## Almond Oil

Almond Oil is rich in Vitamin A, B, and E, which is great for the skin. The Almond Oil helps in maintaining the moisture levels of the skin and gets absorbed quickly without blocking the pores. Almond Oil for skin care helps in improving the complexion, moisturizing, nourishing, relieves dry and irritated skin.

## Jojoba Oil

This oil contains almost all of the vitamins and minerals essential for healthy skin: Vitamin B Complex, Vitamin E, Zinc, Copper, Iodine and Selenium. The oil is even gentle enough to be used on sensitive and delicate skin with reduced chance for allergic reactions. A favorite of massage therapist due to its anti-inflammatory properties. Excellent choice for those who suffer from psoriasis and eczema.

## Neem Oil

This is ideal for acne prone skin because it clears up pimples and removes bacteria that are responsible for causing the break outs. It contains an aspirin like compound which removes the bacteria from the skin, helps to reduce inflammation and redness. The high amount of fatty acid content in Neem Oil prevents and treats scar that occur because of acne. It has been used as a face mask to get rid of the impurities and to tighten the pores.

## Walnut Oil

This oil contains antioxidants such as Gamma Tocopherol and Ellagic Acid which protects cell membranes from harmful effect from outside. Walnut Oil helps the body and skin combat free radicals and reduces the process of aging by prevention of wrinkles and reducing fine lines.

## Apricot Kernel Oil

This oil is a rich source of Oleic Acid and Vitamin E. Both promote healthy skin. This oil is ideal for sensitive skin, prevents premature aging, and penetrates the skin easily. This oil increases energy with its mesmerizing scent, aids in well-being and physical harmony, and balances the nervous system.

## Hazelnut Oil

The presence of Vitamin E, Phytosterols and Stearic Acids helps in treating dry, irritated, damaged, or sensitive skin. It acts as an excellent moisturizer and emollient due to its key essential acids, such as Linoleic Acids. The content of Magnesium, Calcium, and Potassium aids in the oil's natural softening properties and it is often used during massage. Excellent when used regularly and has a slightly nutty scent.

## Grape Seed Oil

The presence of Vitamin E in this oil helps in skin firming and smoothening as it is absorbed easily in the body. It reduces age spots, treats sunburn, and reduces wrinkles and stretch marks. The Linoleic Acid found in this can be very beneficial for treating skin conditions like acne, dermatitis and eczema. The presence of antioxidants in this oil considerably minimizes skin aging. The astringent properties can help tighten the skin. Often used in massage therapy and skin care.

## Olive Oil

Not just for cooking this oil has a slightly olive scent. Although it is thicker in consistency, it is widely used in skin care due to its soothing content of vitamins and minerals.

# THE ESSENTIAL OILS & KEY BENEFITS

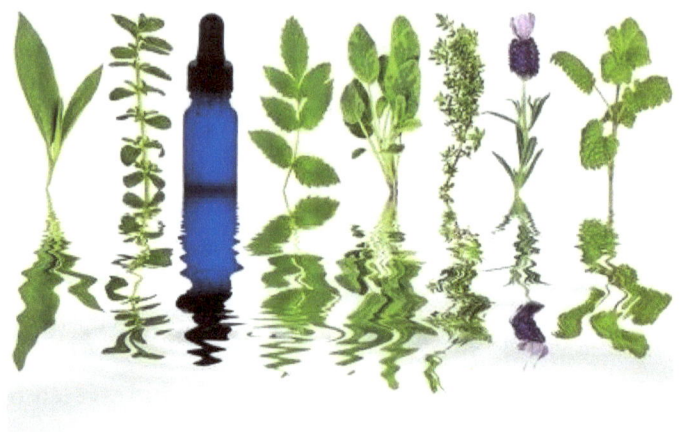

Essential oils are concentrated plant extracts, which are known to contain the essence of the plants. The benefit of using essential oils is their aromatherapy properties that enhance the mind, body, and spirit. Let us have a look at some of the commonly used essential oils used in the preparation of Bath Salts.

## Lavender Oil

It has a beautiful, adaptable fragrance. It is anti-bacterial and a must-have. It's calming and sedative properties makes it a wonderful oil to help relax, combat stress and promote sleep. Lavender Oil is often the first essential oil that is used to help recover from burns. It is also considered safe to use on children's delicate skin.

## Eucalyptus Oil

The benefits of Eucalyptus with its slightly lemony scent include treatment of arthritis, bronchitis, colds, flu, fever, coughing, poor circulation and sinusitis. It is one of the most widely used oils due to its well-known therapeutic properties.

## Rosemary Oil

This oil has a deliciously fresh herb scent and can uplift your mood. Unlike various other oils that contain camphor, this oil is helpful in aching muscles, arthritis, dandruff, dull skin, exhaustion, hair care, muscle cramping, rheumatism.

## Peppermint Oil

The aroma of peppermint is familiar and appealing to most people. It is quite strong and more concentrated than various other types of essential oils. Used by many for the treatment of exhaustion due to its invigorating scent. It has also been known to assist with nausea, colic, congestion, vertigo, muscle sprains, diarrhea, and sinusitis and as an insect repellant.

## Grapefruit Oil

Grapefruit oil is wonderfully energizing oil that isn't too strong or overpowering. As it is rich in vitamins, such as Vitamin C, E, B Complex and K, and minerals. It is often used for the treatment of cellulites, dull skin, toxin build-up, and water retention.

## Rose Oil

With its beautiful scent Rose Oil is known to be helpful during times of anxiety and stress. It is considered the optimal oil for use at the times of grief. It is helpful for insomnia, when used in low concentrations. It is also useful for depression, eczema, mature skin, and most importantly menopause as it provides Gamma-Linoleic Acid that the body requires to make estrogen.

## Tea tree

Tea Tree is an earthy, wood scented oil, used for skin issues. With its antifungal and antibacterial properties it is a must-have oil to keep on hand for a wide array of applications. Use this oil as treatment for acne, cold sores, athlete's foot, cuts, insect bites, itching, dandruff, and psoriasis.

## Vanilla Oil

Vanilla Essential Oil has been used as an antidepressant, sedative, antioxidant, anti-carcinogenic, relaxing and tranquilizing substance. Vanilla Essential Oil stimulates the secretion of testosterone and estrogen which can promote sexual arousal and assist as an aphrodisiac.

## Lemon Oil

Citrus lemon scent has been used to enhance many soaps and scrubs with its happiness inducing aroma. Excellent antiseptic for minor cuts, bites, scraps. It is a natural antihistamine and antiviral and will assist in soothing sore throats, and providing head ache relief when inhaled.

# PREPARATION STORAGE & USE OF BATH SALTS

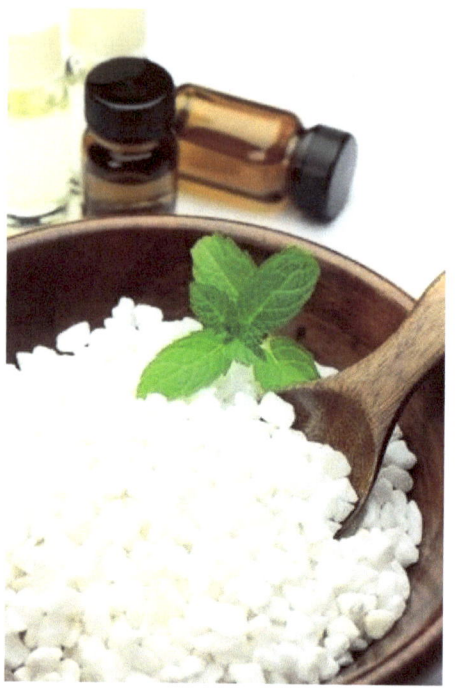

Bath salt recipes can be prepared using one simple method. Storage and use can be drilled down to simplistic detail. Rather than repeat the steps throughout the book, I have placed the methods in this chapter. Simply follow the directions substituting the ingredients from your chosen recipe found in Chapter 5 and the storage method that works best for you and the purpose of the salts.

## Preparing Bath Salts

This is best completed using a large glass bowl. I don't recommend using wood for the bowl, container, or spoons as it can absorb the oils.

1. Measure in a dry measuring cup and avoid mounding in the measuring cup. Use a knife to scrap off excess. 3 cups base salt per batch makes a nice usable quantity. You can use one base salt or mix several. Having different salt size adds a nice touch to the finished product.

2. Place the salts in a large glass mixing bowl.

3. Fold together the salts with either your hand or with a rubber spoon.

**TIP**: Create the salt base in bulk and either store for later or make several recipes at one time. If making several recipes, divide the appropriate portion into individual glass bowls according to the number of different recipes you plan to make.

4. Measure out liquid oils (carrier oil) in liquid measuring cup or measuring spoon.

5. Pour into base salts and fold till well mixed.

6. Scented essential oils are added last to preserve the scent.

**TIP**: I recommend adding the least amount of essential oil drops suggested in the recipe to start. You can always add more, but you can't take the scent away. Play with the concentration until you achieve your desired aroma.

7. Add essential oils, typically 15 - 20 drops to 3 cups of salts is recommended. Add each scent one at a time and mix into the salts till well blended.

**TIP**: If you want your bath salt to have extra pizazz you can add color by using various naturally colored base salts or food colorants. I recommend one drop at a time of food colorants mixed well, or ¼ tsp of mica powder mixed well. Use of colorants can stain your skin, the bath, and cause irritation in those with allergies or sensitive skin. Use colorants sparingly and always read the handling instructions and warnings on the label.

8. Add dried flowers and buds (if indicated and desired) and stir to mix well.

## Storing Bath Salts

Bath salts, when stored in the right container, make excellent useful decor in your bathroom and can create the allusion of a spa just by their presence. In addition, bath salts placed in a decorative container make excellent gifts for any number of occasions.

Storing bath salts in the right manner is essential to the longevity and enjoyment of your salts. If you are like me and tend to make up a large batch at a time, you want to make sure you store them correctly or the scent may have dissipated before you have a chance to use the concoction. Following the steps below will assist in preserving your salts for maximum enjoyment.

1. Use a container that has been properly cleaned and completely dry. Salts can absorb scents, any scents. You do not want to contaminate your delicious salts with the scent or something less than pleasant or a chemical ingredient from something stored in that container prior.

**TIP**: I recommend glass jars or bottles as they will not absorb the scents and oils leaving all the aromatherapy, moisturizing, and healing properties for you to enjoy. Wood can absorb the oils and scents and salts can absorb the scent of metal.

2. Store the prepared bath salts is an air tight container. If moisture gets added to the salt, it gets clumpy or dissolves. Too much humidity and moisture in the air can cause the salts to become hard to work with.

3. Fill disposable cloth bags for individual usage with ½ cup of prepared salt and tightly close bag.

**TIP**: Use of dried flowers and buds add scent and ambiance to your bath. However they do make clean up a little more challenging. I recommend placing these salts in either reusable or disposable bags, found at your local craft store, that allow the salts to dissolve and the flowers to steep. You can make your own if you wish. Just cut pieces of cheese cloth large enough to surround ½ cup of prepared salts, gather ends, and tie or staple shut. You can easily toss a pouch into the bathtub and the salts in it will disperse and dissolve slowly turning the water into a pleasant experience. Then simply toss the flowers that remain in the bag after use. Think tea bags for your tub!

4. Store individual bags for later use in air tight container.

5. Store the ingredients that you will be using in your bath salt recipes in a cool dry place to ensure freshness.

6. Decorative containers can be as simple as canning jars, recycled jam or jelly jars, wine bottles, or small

decorative envelopes or fabric sachet bags. Consider adding a small scoop to the container. Visit your local craft or thrift store and get creative!

## USING BATH SALTS

1. Fill tub to desired level and temperature.

2. Pour ½ cup to 1 cup salts in bath water.  Adding after the water level is achieved will aid in preventing the aroma of the essential oils from evaporating.

3. Allow to dissolve and mix well to disperse the oils and salts.  Sitting on undissolved salts can be uncomfortable!

# SIMPLE BATH SALT RECIPES

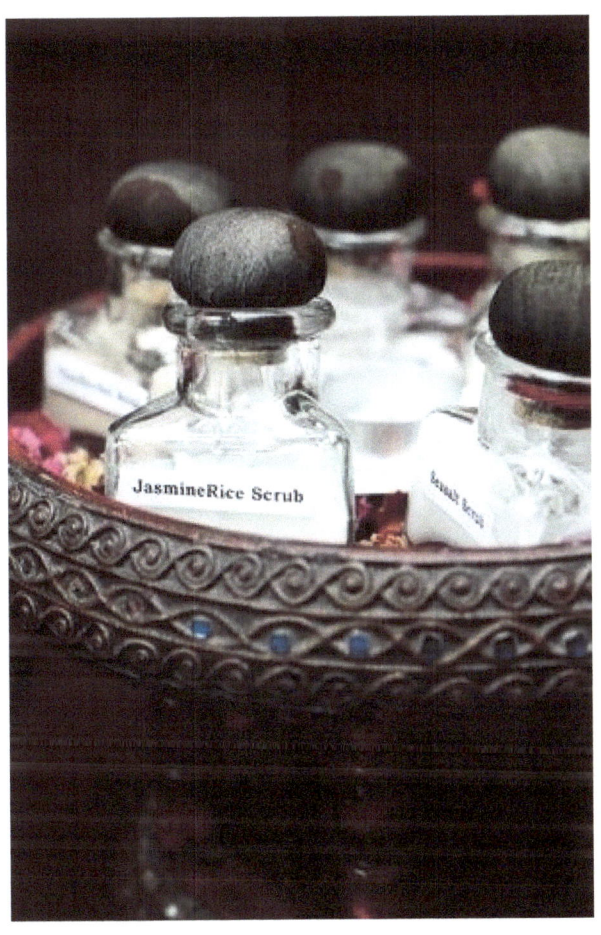

## Glow Salt Recipe

Glow bath salts are generally used as scrub salts. Their perfect combination of avocado and grape oil makes them the preferred recipe for healing dry and wintery skin. The grape oil soothes and provides essential minerals to your skin.

### Ingredients:

- 1 cup Sea Salt

- 1 cup Dead Sea Salt

- 1 cup Avocado Oil

- 1 cup Grape Seed Oil

- 40 - 60 drops Tea Tree Oil

- 4 drops d-alpha Vitamin E

## Neem Chamomile & Dried Flowers

The Neem Chamomile mixture recipe is mostly popular in spa treatments. The anti-bacterial action of the vanilla oil and the medicinal properties of the neem oil make them an ideal choice for killing all kinds of germs on one's body while taking a bath.

## Ingredients:

- 1 cup Sea Salt

- Plastic tea bags or other fine fiber fabric pouch.

- Dried Chamomile Flowers

- 5 drops Neem Oil

- 10 - 15 drops Vanilla Oil

- Dried Lavender Buds

## Salt Scrub by Dead Sea Salts

Salt scrubs are easy to make and Dead Sea Salt scrubs have a number of skin related benefits. One of the biggest benefits is enhancing skin exfoliation and due to their high mineral content. This aids in smoothing skin by removing dead cells.

## Ingredients:

- 2 cups Dead Sea Salt (fine grain)

- 1 cup Almond Oil or Jojoba Oil

- 15  20 drops Essential Oil of your choice

## Crystal Salt

Made from Dead Sea Salt, a very concentrated salt, and Apricot Essential Oil this easily penetrating oil and delicious scent will calm you after a long stressful day. This soothing bath will help to counteract the signs of aging, reduce your aching muscles, and help you sleep.

## Ingredients:

- 1 cup Dead Sea Salt Crystals

- 2 tsps. Apricot Essential Oil

- 5 drops Rose/Rosemary Oil

## Milky Bath Salt

This is a unique recipe as it brilliantly combines the valuable aspects of a milk bath with the goodness of minerals you get from the bath salts and the delicious scent of vanilla and rose. This recipe makes a large quantity of bath salts to store.

## Ingredients:

- 4 cups Sea Salt

- 3 cups Epsom Salt

- 15 drops Rose Essential Oil

- 15 drops Vanilla Essential Oil

- 4 cups Powdered Milk

## Lavender Bath Salt

The calming properties that the Lavender scent elicits is delectable. People normally prepare this Bath Salt by adding various colors and scents. The combination of lavender and rose oil will help you sleep peacefully.

## Ingredients:

- 1 ½ cups Epsom Salt

- 1 ½ cups Sea Salt

- 20 drops Lavender Oil

- 10 drop Rose Oil

# Aromatherapy Pink Bath Salt

This pink salt is beautiful and pure.  Relax with the delicious scent of peppermint and infuse yourself with all the essential vitamins and minerals from the Jojoba Oil while soothing your psoriasis and eczema.

## Ingredients:

- 3 cups Himalayan Pink Salt

- 15 drops Peppermint Oil

- 1 Tbsp. Jojoba Oil

## Vanilla Epsom Bath Salt

This classic Bath Salt can be made with either Epsom Salt or Dead Sea Salt. The Vanilla Oil stimulates the release of testosterone and estrogen and as such can increase sexual arousal.

## Ingredients:

- 1½ cups Epsom Salt

- 7 drops Vanilla Oil

- 1 tsp. Jojoba Oil

# Aromatherapy Almond Bath Salt

Aromatherapy bath salts are a form of alternative medicine as it alters ones cognitive, physical and psychological state of wellbeing.  It is a blend of essential oils with bath salts that turn your bathing time into a skin loving, therapeutic and luxurious experience.

## Ingredients:

- 1 cup Citric Essential Oil

- 5 cups Epsom Salts

- 5 tsps. Sweet Almond Oil

- 2 cup Baking Soda

## Eucalyptus Bath Salts

Scented bath salts are popular for creating a scented ambiance in your bath. The mix of the essential oils and vegetable oils provide you a silky and luxurious experience. Eucalyptus also acts as a deodorant while the Epsom salt eases stress and relaxes your body.

## Ingredients:

- 2 tsps. liquid oil of your choice (jojoba, almond, apricot, olive)

- 5 – 10 drops Eucalyptus Oil

- 2 cups Epsom Salt

- Optional: ¼ cup Sea Salt

## Energizer Bath Salt

Energizer bath salts are a result of a proportionate mixture of peppermint and rosemary oil. The combination of these essential oils with Epsom Salt has a number of health benefits like body pain reduction and healing of sprains and bruises.

## Ingredients:

- 1 cup Sea Salt

- 2 cups Epsom Salt

- 10 drops Rosemary Oil

- 6 drops Eucalyptus Oil

- 15 drops Peppermint Oil

## Back Pain Relaxing Bath Salts

Soaking in the Epsom Salt is known as the king of remedies, particularly for sore muscles. This is because the Magnesium Sulphate present in Epsom Salt is readily absorbed for quick relief of inflammation.

## Ingredients:

- 1½ cups Epsom Salt

- ¾ cup Bi-Carb Soda

- 10 drops Peppermint Oil

- 5 drops Rosemary Oil

- 5 drops Lavender Oil

- 5 drops Eucalyptus Oil

- 1 Tbsp. Rosemary fresh sprigs

- 1 Tbsp. Lavender flowers (dried)

# Before you go…..

Thank you again for choosing *Bath Salts Basics.* There is no time like the present to get started with learning how to make your own homemade salts. The recipes mentioned in the book are easy to prepare, allowing you to create a delightful healing bathing experience in the comfort of your own home.

In today's modern life, most of us are so busy that we often neglect our skin care and due to time constraints we prefer to pick up most of our health care items from the beauty stores. Why not add a little creativity to these brilliant salts and oils and make our own bath salts at home?

If you have ever experienced a luxury spa or a bath and wish to pamper yourself, this guide is definitely going to take you to the next level where you can set the moods using your own preferred fragrances, as you prepare the natural soothing bath salts at home.

It is my hope that this book gave you the tools needed and the confidence to start creating your own salts tailored to your current needs and desires. Perhaps inspire you to get creative and venture farther into the art of making delicious salts.

Why not share your creations with a homemade gift of healing salts for those special people in your life. Easy to make in bulk, you can create your own and have enough left over to gift to others.

How about enchanting:

- Your child's teacher at school.

- A bride to be at her shower or bachelorette bash.

- Your bridal party or wedding guests.

- Your coworkers or boss.

- A new neighbor as a welcome and an ice breaker into conversation.

- Someone who has gone above and beyond in a special way for you.

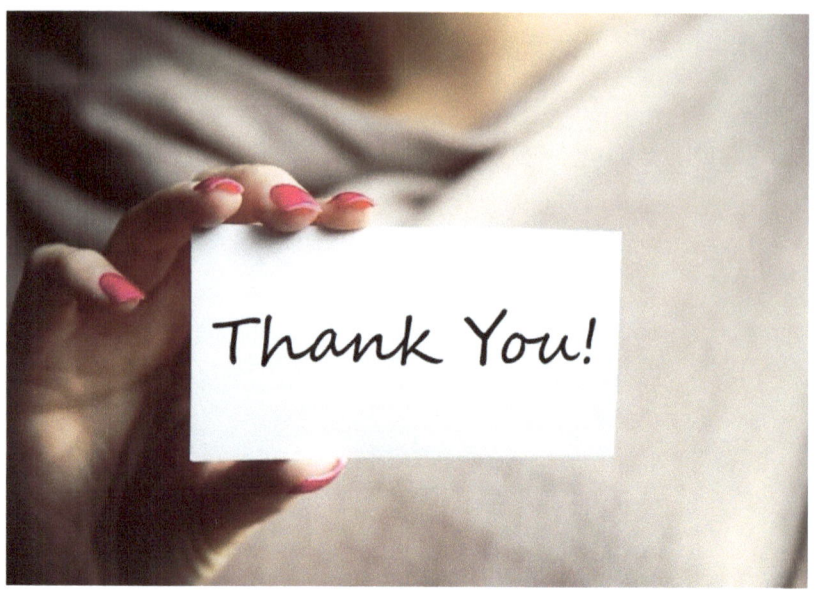

May I ask one more thing? I would be most grateful if you would leave a review on Amazon. This will help others when making their selection. If you haven't yet taken advantage of my free gift, please return to the front page and do so before leaving.

From my home to yours,

*Stella*

**Check out our other books currently available on Amazon:**

*Pegan Central: Smoothies & Juices for Super Health*

*Pegan Central: The Pegan Recipe Book*

*Vegan One Pot Cookbook: Delicious Easy Recipes for Healthy Eating*

*Skinny Bottoms Up: Easy Guilt Free Low Sugar Holiday Cocktails*

*Kidz Treats; Gluten Egg Peanut Dairy Free Recipe Makeovers*

*Pie Lovers Cookbook: Delicious Quick and Easy Recipes For Newbies to Foodies*

*Comfort Food: Quick & Easy Gluten and Dairy Free Recipes*

*Body Butter Basics: Easy Guide to Homemade Body Butters, Including Simple Recipes*

And coming soon...

Caveman Man Cave

www.ingramcontent.com/pod-product-compliance
Lightning Source LLC
Chambersburg PA
CBHW050839290526
45792CB00001B/463